Ashley Fitzgerald

FOOD THERAPY
FOR
HEMORRHOIDS
The Healing Power of Food

Published by UNITEXTO

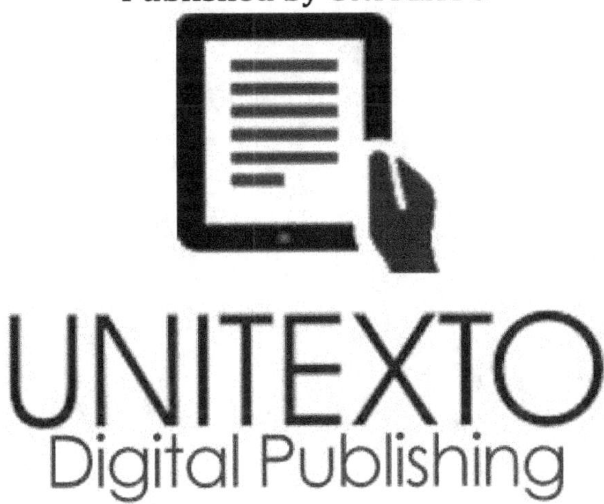

Table of Contents

Why this book?

Welcome to "Food Therapy for Hemorrhoids," a guide that opens a new chapter in your journey towards health and wellness. This book is born out of the understanding that the foods we consume play a crucial role in not just our general health but in managing specific conditions like hemorrhoids. In these pages, you will discover a holistic approach to soothing and preventing hemorrhoid flare-ups through dietary choices.

Hemorrhoids, a common yet seldom discussed ailment, affect a significant portion of the population. Often associated with discomfort and pain, this condition can be a source of significant distress. Traditional treatments range from over-the-counter solutions to surgical interventions, but these methods often overlook a critical component of health: nutrition.

In recent years, there has been a growing recognition of the role diet plays in managing various health conditions. "Food Therapy for Hemorrhoids" is at the forefront of this movement, offering a comprehensive guide to understanding how certain foods can alleviate, and even prevent, the symptoms of hemorrhoids.

The book begins by exploring the basics of hemorrhoids: what they are, why they occur, and the common triggers that can cause flare-ups. This foundational knowledge is crucial for anyone looking to manage their condition effectively.

From there, we delve into the heart of the matter: the relationship between diet and hemorrhoids. You'll learn about the importance of fiber in maintaining digestive health, the role of hydration, and how certain foods can reduce inflammation and promote healing. This isn't just a list of foods to eat and avoid; it's an exploration of how and why these foods impact your body.

One of the core principles of this book is that dietary changes should be sustainable and enjoyable. To that end, we provide practical advice on incorporating these food recommendations into your daily life. You'll find tips for meal planning, grocery shopping, and making gradual changes to your diet.

The book also addresses common misconceptions and challenges that people face when adjusting their diet. We understand that change isn't always easy, and our goal is to support you through each step of this journey.

A highlight of "Food Therapy for Hemorrhoids" is the collection of recipes designed specifically for individuals dealing with hemorrhoids. These recipes aren't just healthy and beneficial for your condition; they're also delicious and varied, ensuring that you enjoy your meals while nurturing your body.

As we progress, the book also touches upon the importance of other lifestyle factors, such as exercise and stress management, in conjunction with a balanced diet. The holistic approach ensures that you're not just treating symptoms but enhancing your overall quality of life.

In the final chapters, we offer guidance on maintaining these dietary and lifestyle changes long-term. This isn't just a temporary fix; it's a way of life. The book concludes with inspirational stories from individuals who have successfully managed their hemorrhoids through dietary changes, offering hope and motivation.

"Food Therapy for Hemorrhoids" is more than just a book; it's a companion on your path to better health. It empowers you

with knowledge, guides you with practical advice, and supports you with a community of people who share your journey.
As you turn these pages, we invite you to open your mind to the possibility of healing and comfort through the foods you eat.

Welcome to a new way of living, where your diet is your ally in health, and every meal brings you one step closer to relief and well-being.

Ashley Fitzgerald

About the Author

Ashley Fitzgerald: An Embodiment of Healing and Personal Triumph
From a tender age, I, Ashley Fitzgerald, was acutely attuned to the nuances of health and personal well-being. These early inklings of self-awareness were not just passing contemplations but the seeds of a lifelong journey towards self-improvement and healing. As the chapters of life unfolded, I embraced my calling with fervor, transforming my youthful concerns into a robust career that spans two decades.

Today, I stand before you not merely as a practitioner but as a seasoned professional healer whose hands and heart have been instrumental in guiding countless individuals towards weight loss triumphs, enriched sexual health, and the surmounting of life's multifaceted challenges to reach the pinnacle of their health aspirations.

My professional and academic journey is a tapestry of diverse yet interconnected disciplines. With an insatiable thirst for knowledge, I delved deep into the realms of yoga and meditation, not just as practices but as academic pursuits, seeking to understand their profound effects on the human psyche and physiology.

This spiritual and intellectual quest further led me to the healing energies of Reiki, the organic wisdom in health foods, and the transformative potential of neuroscience and positive psychology. My foray into the science of health and exercise is not merely academic; it is a reflection of my intrinsic philosophy that the body and mind are inextricable partners in the dance of life.

My dedication to personal growth extends beyond my professional endeavors—it is a way of life. Each morning, as the world stirs awake, I find sanctuary in my daily rituals. My practice of yoga is more than a physical regimen; it is a journey towards achieving a state of zen-like tranquility, a testament to my belief in the power of simplicity and inner peace. Meditation accompanies yoga as my mental compass, guiding me through life's tumultuous waves with a steadfast calm.

What fuels my unyielding passion is an unwavering drive—an innate desire to not only absorb the myriad teachings that life has to offer but also to disseminate them. I am imbued with a relentless drive to unearth and share life strategies that spark a transformative flame within souls, urging them to reach for health, well-being, and the fruition of their deepest dreams.

It was this very desire that led me to the world of writing, to become a scribe of my experiences and insights. My pen is driven by a profound commitment to be a beacon of positivity, influencing the lives of others through words that resonate with truth and vitality.

As you turn the pages of my books, what you will find is a reflection of my heart's work. I invite you into my world, not just as a reader, but as a fellow traveler on this grand adventure of life.

Thank you for embarking on this journey with me, and it is my sincerest hope that you will find as much joy in reading my writings as I found in penning them down. May the words you peruse inspire you to cultivate the health and happiness you so richly deserve.

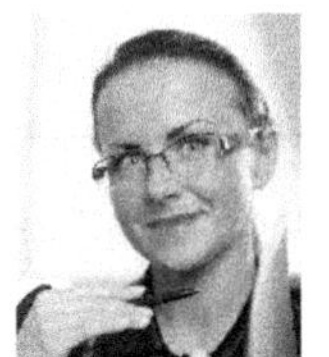

Ashley Fitzgerald

Chapter 1: Introduction to Hemorrhoids

Understanding Hemorrhoids: Causes and Symptoms

Hemorrhoids, commonly known as piles, are swollen veins in the lower rectum and anus, similar to varicose veins. They can develop inside the rectum (internal hemorrhoids) or under the skin around the anus (external hemorrhoids). The exact cause of hemorrhoids is often unknown, but they are associated with increased pressure in the lower rectum due to straining during bowel movements, prolonged sitting, chronic constipation or diarrhea, obesity, and pregnancy.

Symptoms of hemorrhoids include pain, discomfort, itching, swelling, and bleeding during bowel movements. In some cases, an external hemorrhoid may develop a clot (thrombosis), leading to severe pain, inflammation, and a hard lump near the anus.

The Role of Diet in Hemorrhoid Management

Diet plays a crucial role in the management and prevention of hemorrhoids. A diet high in fiber can soften the stool and increase its bulk, which helps to reduce straining during bowel movements. Adequate hydration is also essential to prevent constipation and reduce pressure on hemorrhoids.

Case Study: John's Journey with Hemorrhoids

John, a 45-year-old office worker, had been suffering from painful hemorrhoids for several months. His sedentary lifestyle and low-fiber diet contributed to severe constipation, exacerbating his condition. After several painful episodes, John decided to seek medical advice.

His doctor recommended a dietary overhaul, focusing on high-fiber foods like whole grains, vegetables, and fruits, along with increased fluid intake. Within weeks of making these changes, John noticed a significant reduction in pain and discomfort. His bowel movements became more regular, and the swelling reduced considerably.

John's story highlights the impact of diet on hemorrhoid management and the importance of lifestyle changes in alleviating symptoms.

Expert Interview: Dietary Recommendations from a Gastroenterologist

Dr. Emily Chen, a renowned gastroenterologist, emphasizes the importance of diet in managing hemorrhoids. "The first line of defense against hemorrhoids is often a dietary change," she explains. "A diet rich in fiber can significantly reduce the symptoms and even prevent the occurrence of hemorrhoids."

Dr. Chen recommends incorporating a variety of fiber-rich foods into the diet, such as legumes, whole grains, fruits, and vegetables. She also stresses the importance of hydration. "Drinking plenty of water is essential. It helps in softening the stool and ensures smooth bowel movements," she adds.

For patients resistant to dietary changes, Dr. Chen suggests starting with small, incremental changes, like adding a serving of vegetables to each meal or replacing white bread with whole grain alternatives.

Real-Life Story: Maria's Battle with Postpartum Hemorrhoids

After giving birth to her first child, Maria developed painful external hemorrhoids, a common occurrence in postpartum women. The discomfort made it difficult for her to care for her newborn.

Maria's midwife suggested increasing her fiber intake and staying well-hydrated. She started her day with a high-fiber cereal, snacked on fruits like pears and oranges, and included salads and steamed vegetables in her meals. She also made a conscious effort to drink at least eight glasses of water a day.

These dietary changes, coupled with regular light exercise, helped Maria manage her symptoms effectively. Within a few weeks, she experienced significant relief, which allowed her to focus better on her newborn.

Conclusion

Hemorrhoids are a common yet uncomfortable condition that can significantly impact a person's quality of life. The case studies and expert opinions in this chapter underscore the critical role of diet in managing hemorrhoid symptoms. A diet rich in fiber, coupled with adequate hydration, can ease the symptoms and may even prevent the development of hemorrhoids.

For individuals like John and Maria, simple dietary adjustments made a significant difference in their comfort and ability to manage hemorrhoids. As Dr. Chen suggests, these dietary changes, along with a healthy lifestyle, can be a first line of defense against the discomfort caused by hemorrhoids.

Understanding the causes and symptoms of hemorrhoids is the first step toward effective management. With the right dietary approach, many individuals can find relief from this common condition.

Chapter 2: The Importance of Fiber

Types of Fiber: Soluble vs. Insoluble

Fiber is an essential component of a healthy diet, especially for individuals with hemorrhoids. It is broadly classified into two types: soluble and insoluble. Soluble fiber dissolves in water to form a gel-like substance, aiding in digestion and helping to soften the stool. Sources include oats, legumes, apples, and blueberries. Insoluble fiber, on the other hand, does not dissolve in water and helps add bulk to the stool, preventing constipation. Good sources are whole grains, nuts, and many vegetables.

Both types of fiber are important for hemorrhoid management, as they facilitate easier bowel movements and reduce the strain that can exacerbate hemorrhoid symptoms.

High-Fiber Foods for Hemorrhoid Relief

Incorporating high-fiber foods into the diet is crucial for hemorrhoid relief. Foods such as bran cereals, beans, lentils, fruits, and vegetables are excellent choices. These foods not only help in regulating bowel movements but also play a role in overall digestive health.

Case Study: Alex's High-Fiber Diet Transformation

Alex, a 30-year-old software engineer, suffered from chronic hemorrhoids. His diet mainly consisted of processed foods with minimal fiber content. This dietary habit led to regular constipation and painful hemorrhoid flare-ups.

After consulting a dietician, Alex began incorporating more high-fiber foods into his diet. He started his day with a bowl of bran cereal and included more fruits and vegetables in his meals. Snacks consisted of nuts and whole-grain crackers instead of chips and cookies. These changes led to a marked improvement in his bowel habits and a significant reduction in hemorrhoid pain and discomfort.

Alex's experience demonstrates the importance of a high-fiber diet in managing hemorrhoids effectively.

Expert Interview: Nutritional Advice from a Dietitian

Sarah Thompson, a registered dietitian, emphasizes the importance of a balanced diet rich in both types of fiber. "Many people underestimate the power of fiber in preventing and managing hemorrhoids," she states. "A balanced intake of both soluble and insoluble fiber is key. Soluble fiber softens the stool, while insoluble fiber helps it pass more easily."

Sarah recommends aiming for 25-30 grams of fiber per day. She advises her clients to start slowly when introducing more fiber to avoid bloating and to drink plenty of water to help fiber work more effectively.

Real-Life Story: Linda's Recovery from Hemorrhoids Through Diet

Linda, a 55-year-old teacher, struggled with hemorrhoids for years. Despite trying various treatments, she found little relief until she changed her diet. With the guidance of a nutritionist, Linda started to incorporate a variety of high-fiber foods into her diet. She replaced white bread with whole grain bread, included more legumes in her meals, and snacked on fruits like pears and apples.

These dietary changes, combined with increased water intake, greatly improved her symptoms. Linda noticed softer stools, less straining during bowel movements, and a significant reduction in hemorrhoid discomfort.

Linda's story is a testament to how dietary changes can effectively manage hemorrhoids.

Conclusion

The role of fiber in the diet cannot be overstated, especially for those suffering from hemorrhoids. As illustrated by the experiences of Alex and Linda, incorporating a variety of high-fiber foods can lead to significant improvements in symptoms. The insights provided by experts like Sarah Thompson further highlight the importance of a balanced fiber intake for digestive health and hemorrhoid management.

Understanding the different types of fiber and how they contribute to bowel health is the first step in adjusting one's diet for hemorrhoid relief. As we have seen, making these changes can lead to a marked improvement in symptoms, offering a natural and effective way to manage this common condition.

Chapter 3: Hydration and Hemorrhoids

The Role of Water in Digestive Health

Water is a fundamental component of digestive health, playing a critical role in the prevention and management of hemorrhoids. Adequate hydration helps to soften the stool, making bowel movements easier and reducing the strain that can lead to hemorrhoids or exacerbate existing ones. Water also aids in digestion and the absorption of nutrients, ensuring the smooth functioning of the gastrointestinal system.

Hydration Tips for Hemorrhoid Sufferers

For individuals suffering from hemorrhoids, staying well-hydrated is crucial. It's recommended to drink at least eight 8-ounce glasses of water daily, although needs can vary based on individual factors like activity level and climate. Incorporating water-rich foods like cucumbers, watermelons, and oranges can also contribute to overall hydration.

Case Study: Michael's Hydration-Focused Recovery

Michael, a 40-year-old construction worker, often neglected his water intake due to the nature of his job. Suffering from persistent hemorrhoids, he experienced significant discomfort, particularly during bowel movements.

His doctor advised him to prioritize hydration as part of his treatment plan. Michael started carrying a water bottle with him at all times, ensuring he drank regularly throughout the day. He also increased his intake of fruits and vegetables with high water content. These changes resulted in softer stools and less strain during bowel movements, providing considerable relief from his hemorrhoid symptoms.

Michael's story underscores the importance of hydration in managing hemorrhoids, particularly for individuals in physically demanding jobs.

Expert Interview: Insights from a Gastroenterologist

Dr. Angela Richardson, a gastroenterologist with extensive experience treating hemorrhoid patients, emphasizes the importance of hydration. "Water is often overlooked in digestive health," she notes. "For hemorrhoid sufferers, it's not just about eating the right foods. Staying adequately hydrated is equally important."

Dr. Richardson advises against excessive caffeine and alcohol, as they can lead to dehydration. She recommends herbal teas and infusing water with fruits for those who struggle with plain water. "It's about making hydration a regular part of your routine," she adds.

Real-Life Story: Emma's Lifestyle Change

Emma, a 50-year-old librarian, had chronic hemorrhoids exacerbated by her sedentary job and poor hydration habits. After a particularly painful flare-up, she decided to make a change.

She began tracking her water intake and set reminders to drink water throughout the day. Emma also swapped her afternoon coffee for herbal tea and increased her consumption of water-rich fruits and vegetables. These adjustments led to a noticeable improvement in her bowel habits and a significant decrease in hemorrhoid discomfort.

Emma's experience demonstrates the impact of simple lifestyle changes on hemorrhoid management.

Conclusion

Hydration plays a vital role in the management of hemorrhoids, as evidenced by the experiences of individuals like Michael and Emma. The expert insights provided by Dr. Richardson further highlight the necessity of maintaining adequate hydration for digestive health and hemorrhoid relief.

Ensuring proper hydration can soften stools, reduce straining during bowel movements, and aid in overall digestive function, offering a practical and accessible method for managing hemorrhoids. As this chapter illustrates, incorporating sufficient water intake into one's daily routine, along with mindful dietary choices, can lead to substantial improvements in hemorrhoid symptoms and overall well-being.

Chapter 4: Anti-Inflammatory Foods

Foods That Reduce Inflammation

Inflammation is a significant factor in many health conditions, including hemorrhoids. An anti-inflammatory diet focuses on foods that can help reduce inflammation and alleviate the symptoms associated with hemorrhoids. These foods are rich in antioxidants, omega-3 fatty acids, and other nutrients that support overall health and reduce inflammation. Key components of such a diet include leafy green vegetables, fatty fish like salmon, nuts, seeds, and whole grains.

Creating an Anti-Inflammatory Diet Plan

Creating an anti-inflammatory diet plan involves incorporating a variety of these foods into daily meals while avoiding or reducing intake of foods that can exacerbate inflammation, such as processed foods, excessive sugar, and certain types of fats.

Case Study: Rachel's Recovery with an Anti-Inflammatory Diet

Rachel, a 35-year-old graphic designer, had been suffering from persistent hemorrhoids for several months. After researching various remedies, she came across the concept of an anti-inflammatory diet. Determined to find relief, Rachel began incorporating more anti-inflammatory foods into her meals.

She started her day with a smoothie made from spinach, berries, and flaxseeds, and snacked on nuts instead of processed snacks. Her lunches and dinners consisted of lean proteins, whole grains, and plenty of vegetables. Within a few weeks, Rachel noticed a significant improvement in her symptoms. Her hemorrhoids became less painful, and her overall health improved.

Expert Interview: Nutritional Advice from a Dietitian

Melanie Johnson, a registered dietitian specializing in anti-inflammatory diets, emphasizes the importance of such diets in managing conditions like hemorrhoids. "An anti-inflammatory diet can be a game-changer for many of my clients," Melanie says. "It's about more than just reducing symptoms; it's about improving overall health."

Melanie recommends a diet rich in fruits and vegetables, whole grains, lean protein, and healthy fats. She advises her clients to be mindful of their intake of refined sugars and processed foods. "Small changes can lead to big results," Melanie adds, emphasizing the need for a balanced approach.

Real-Life Story: David's Transformation

David, a 50-year-old school principal, struggled with hemorrhoids for years. After a particularly severe flare-up, he sought advice from a nutritionist, who recommended an anti-inflammatory diet. David was skeptical but decided to give it a try.

He replaced red meat with fatty fish like salmon and mackerel, increased his intake of fruits and vegetables, and started using olive oil for cooking instead of butter. He also cut down on sugary snacks and processed foods. The changes weren't easy, but within a couple of months, David felt a noticeable difference. His hemorrhoids were less bothersome, and he had more energy and less digestive discomfort.

Conclusion

The incorporation of anti-inflammatory foods into the diet can have a profound impact on the management of hemorrhoids, as seen in the experiences of Rachel and David. The guidance provided by dietitians like Melanie Johnson further highlights the role of diet in reducing inflammation and managing symptoms.

An anti-inflammatory diet is not just beneficial for hemorrhoids but also contributes to overall health and well-being. It demonstrates the power of food as medicine, offering a natural and holistic approach to health care. This chapter underscores the significance of dietary choices in managing conditions like hemorrhoids and the broader implications for long-term health.

Chapter 5: Gut Health and Probiotics

The Link Between Gut Health and Hemorrhoids

Gut health is increasingly recognized as a key factor in overall well-being, including the management of conditions like hemorrhoids. A healthy gut flora aids in digestion, nutrient absorption, and bowel regularity, all of which are crucial in preventing and managing hemorrhoids. An imbalance in gut bacteria can lead to issues like constipation or diarrhea, exacerbating hemorrhoid symptoms.

Probiotic Foods and Supplements

Probiotics are live bacteria and yeasts that are beneficial for gut health. They are found in fermented foods like yogurt, kefir, sauerkraut, and kombucha, as well as in supplement form. Incorporating probiotics into the diet can help maintain a healthy balance of gut bacteria, aiding in digestion and potentially alleviating hemorrhoid symptoms.

Case Study: Emily's Journey to Better Gut Health

Emily, a 28-year-old yoga instructor, suffered from chronic constipation and hemorrhoids. Her discomfort led her to explore various dietary changes. After learning about the benefits of probiotics, Emily began incorporating more probiotic-rich foods into her diet. She started her day with Greek yogurt, added sauerkraut to her meals, and regularly drank kombucha.

Additionally, Emily took a daily probiotic supplement on her doctor's recommendation. Over time, she noticed an improvement in her bowel habits and a decrease in hemorrhoid flare-ups. Emily's experience highlights the potential benefits of probiotics for individuals suffering from hemorrhoids.

Expert Interview: Insights from a Gastroenterologist

Dr. Lucas Nguyen, a gastroenterologist specializing in digestive disorders, explains the connection between gut health and hemorrhoids. "The gut microbiome plays a vital role in digestive health. A balanced microbiome can help prevent constipation, a major contributing factor to hemorrhoids," he says.

Dr. Nguyen recommends incorporating a variety of probiotic-rich foods into the diet for their potential benefits. "While research is still ongoing, there's promising evidence that probiotics can aid in managing digestive issues, including those that lead to hemorrhoids," he adds.

Real-Life Story: Mark's Transformation with Probiotics

Mark, a 45-year-old truck driver, faced challenges managing his hemorrhoids due to his sedentary job and irregular eating habits. After a particularly painful episode, Mark sought advice from a nutritionist, who suggested adding probiotics to his diet.

He began consuming yogurt daily and added fermented foods like kimchi to his meals. Mark also started taking a probiotic supplement. These changes, combined with increased water intake and dietary fiber, led to improved bowel movements and significant relief from his hemorrhoid symptoms.

Mark's story demonstrates the impact of probiotics on gut health and, consequently, on the management of hemorrhoids.

Conclusion

The relationship between gut health and hemorrhoids is an important aspect of managing this condition. As shown in the experiences of Emily and Mark, incorporating probiotics into the diet can have a positive impact on digestive health and hemorrhoid management. The insights provided by experts like Dr. Nguyen highlight the potential of probiotics as a complementary approach to traditional hemorrhoid treatments.

Focusing on gut health through the inclusion of probiotic foods and supplements can offer a natural and effective way to improve bowel habits and alleviate the symptoms associated with hemorrhoids. This chapter underscores the importance of a holistic approach to health, where dietary choices play a crucial role in managing and preventing conditions like hemorrhoids.

Chapter 6: Foods to Avoid

Identifying Trigger Foods for Hemorrhoids

Diet plays a significant role in the management of hemorrhoids, and certain foods can exacerbate the condition. Common trigger foods include those high in refined sugars, fats, and certain spices. These can contribute to constipation or diarrhea, worsening hemorrhoid symptoms. Identifying and avoiding these triggers is crucial for individuals suffering from this condition.

Strategies for Dietary Modification

Modifying one's diet to manage hemorrhoids involves not only adding beneficial foods but also removing or reducing the intake of certain foods. This requires a mindful approach to eating, paying attention to how different foods affect one's body and symptoms.

Case Study: Anna's Elimination Diet

Anna, a 38-year-old teacher, struggled with hemorrhoids for years. Her diet was rich in processed foods, and she often experienced severe hemorrhoid flare-ups. After consulting with a nutritionist, Anna decided to try an elimination diet to identify her trigger foods.

She started by removing processed foods, particularly those high in refined sugars and unhealthy fats, from her diet. She also reduced her intake of spicy foods, which she noticed often exacerbated her symptoms. Over several weeks, Anna reintroduced foods one at a time, noting any changes in her symptoms.

This process helped Anna identify specific foods that worsened her hemorrhoids. By avoiding these triggers, she experienced a significant decrease in pain and discomfort.

Expert Interview: Dietary Advice from a Nutritionist

Julie Chen, a certified nutritionist, emphasizes the importance of avoiding trigger foods for hemorrhoid sufferers. "Each individual's triggers may be different, but there are common culprits like spicy foods, alcohol, caffeine, and processed foods that can exacerbate symptoms," she explains.

Julie advises her clients to keep a food diary to track what they eat and how it affects their symptoms. "Awareness is the first step towards change. By understanding which foods worsen your symptoms, you can make more informed dietary choices," she adds.

Real-Life Story: Michael's Journey to a Hemorrhoid-Friendly Diet

Michael, a 50-year-old software developer, had chronic hemorrhoids. Despite various treatments, he found little relief until he addressed his diet. Under the guidance of a dietitian, Michael learned that his love for spicy foods and coffee was contributing to his condition.

He gradually reduced his intake of these items, replacing them with healthier alternatives. Michael also cut back on alcohol and started focusing on a diet rich in fiber and hydration. These changes not only alleviated his hemorrhoid symptoms but also improved his overall digestive health.

Conclusion

Identifying and avoiding trigger foods is an essential aspect of managing hemorrhoids. As demonstrated in the experiences of Anna and Michael, dietary modifications can lead to significant improvements in symptoms. Expert insights from nutritionists like Julie Chen provide valuable guidance on how to approach these dietary changes.

Through careful observation and adjustments, individuals suffering from hemorrhoids can identify their specific dietary triggers and make the necessary changes to alleviate their symptoms. This chapter highlights the importance of a personalized approach to diet, one that is mindful of the unique needs and reactions of each individual in managing hemorrhoids.

Chapter 7: Meal Planning and Preparation

Creating Hemorrhoid-Friendly Meal Plans

Effectively managing hemorrhoids often involves dietary changes. Creating hemorrhoid-friendly meal plans means incorporating foods that are high in fiber, low in inflammatory agents, and gentle on the digestive system. Such meal plans should aim to reduce symptoms like constipation and inflammation, common triggers for hemorrhoid discomfort.

Easy and Nutritious Recipes

The key to sticking to a hemorrhoid-friendly diet is having a variety of easy and nutritious recipes. These recipes should focus on whole foods, be rich in fiber, and include ingredients known for their anti-inflammatory properties.

Case Study: Sarah's Weekly Meal Prep

Sarah, a 42-year-old accountant and mother of two, struggled to manage her hemorrhoid symptoms while balancing a busy schedule. She found that meal planning and preparation were crucial in maintaining a diet that helped manage her condition.

Each Sunday, Sarah dedicated a few hours to preparing meals for the week. She focused on high-fiber foods like lentils, quinoa, and a variety of vegetables. She made large batches of soups and stews that were easy to reheat and packed with nutrients. This preparation not only helped her manage her symptoms but also saved her time during the hectic workweek.

Expert Interview: Nutritional Guidance from a Chef

Chef David Martinez, known for his focus on healthy cuisine, offers valuable insights into preparing hemorrhoid-friendly meals. "Cooking for health doesn't have to be bland or boring," he says. "The key is using fresh ingredients and herbs to enhance flavor without adding irritants like excessive spices or fats."

Chef Martinez recommends recipes like grilled salmon with steamed vegetables, quinoa salads with fresh herbs, and fruit smoothies with spinach and flaxseeds. "These meals are not only nutritious but also help in managing digestive health," he adds.

Real-Life Story: Tom's Culinary Journey

Tom, a 35-year-old freelance writer, found his hemorrhoid symptoms worsening due to poor eating habits. With limited cooking skills, he often opted for takeout, which usually meant unhealthy choices. Determined to change his diet, Tom started learning simple, nutritious recipes.

He began with easy dishes like oatmeal with berries for breakfast and grilled chicken with a side of mixed vegetables for dinner. He explored cooking with legumes and whole grains, creating hearty salads and stir-fries. Over time, Tom's cooking skills improved, as did his hemorrhoid symptoms, illustrating the power of diet in managing this condition.

Conclusion

Creating and adhering to a hemorrhoid-friendly meal plan is a crucial step in managing symptoms. As seen in the experiences of Sarah and Tom, preparing nutritious meals that focus on fiber and anti-inflammatory ingredients can significantly alleviate discomfort caused by hemorrhoids.

The advice from experts like Chef Martinez highlights the importance of flavorful, health-focused cooking. By embracing meal planning and preparation, individuals suffering from hemorrhoids can not only manage their symptoms more effectively but also enjoy a diverse and satisfying diet. This chapter underscores the role of dietary choices in controlling hemorrhoid symptoms and the value of investing time in preparing healthful meals.

Chapter 8: Lifestyle and Dietary Habits

The Impact of Lifestyle on Hemorrhoids

Hemorrhoids are not only influenced by diet but also by overall lifestyle habits. Factors such as physical activity, stress management, and eating patterns play a significant role in the development and management of this condition. A sedentary lifestyle, high-stress levels, and irregular eating habits can exacerbate hemorrhoid symptoms, while a balanced lifestyle can help mitigate them.

Incorporating Healthy Eating Habits

Adopting healthy eating habits is crucial for managing hemorrhoids. This includes eating meals at regular intervals, consuming a balanced diet rich in fiber, and staying hydrated. It also involves mindful eating practices, such as chewing food thoroughly and eating in a relaxed environment.

Case Study: Lisa's Lifestyle Overhaul

Lisa, a 40-year-old marketing executive, suffered from severe hemorrhoids, exacerbated by her high-stress job and sedentary lifestyle. Her erratic eating patterns and reliance on fast food contributed to her condition. After a particularly painful flare-up, Lisa knew she needed to make a change.

She started by incorporating regular exercise into her routine, focusing on activities like walking and yoga, which improved her circulation and digestion. She also made an effort to eat more mindfully, setting aside time for balanced, home-cooked meals. These lifestyle changes, along with better stress management, led to a noticeable improvement in her hemorrhoid symptoms.

Expert Interview: Lifestyle Recommendations from a Health Coach

Grace Kim, a health coach specializing in digestive health, discusses the importance of holistic lifestyle changes for managing hemorrhoids. "It's not just about what you eat, but also how and when you eat," Grace explains. "Regular physical activity, stress reduction, and structured meal times are all important."

Grace advises her clients to find physical activities they enjoy, which makes regular exercise more sustainable. She also recommends techniques like meditation or deep breathing for stress management. "These practices can have a profound impact on your digestive health and, consequently, hemorrhoids," she adds.

Real-Life Story: Kevin's Transformation

Kevin, a 55-year-old teacher, had long-standing issues with hemorrhoids, partly due to his inactive lifestyle and poor dietary habits. After his condition worsened, he decided to take action. Kevin revamped his diet, focusing on high-fiber foods and eliminating processed foods. He also started a moderate exercise regimen and took up meditation to manage stress.

These changes didn't just alleviate his hemorrhoid symptoms; they also improved his overall quality of life. Kevin experienced increased energy levels, better sleep, and a more positive outlook on life.

Conclusion

Lifestyle factors play a significant role in the management of hemorrhoids, as demonstrated by Lisa and Kevin's experiences. The guidance provided by experts like Grace Kim emphasizes the importance of a holistic approach, incorporating not only dietary changes but also physical activity and stress management.

Adopting a lifestyle that supports digestive health can significantly reduce the symptoms of hemorrhoids and enhance overall well-being. This chapter highlights the interconnectedness of various lifestyle aspects with hemorrhoid management, underscoring the importance of comprehensive lifestyle changes in addressing this condition.

Chapter 9: Supplements and Natural Remedies

Supplements for Hemorrhoid Relief

In addition to dietary and lifestyle changes, supplements can play a role in managing hemorrhoid symptoms. Common supplements for hemorrhoid relief include fiber supplements, flavonoids, and omega-3 fatty acids, which can help reduce inflammation, improve bowel movements, and strengthen blood vessels.

Herbal Remedies and Their Efficacy

Herbal remedies have been used for centuries to treat various ailments, including hemorrhoids. Herbs such as witch hazel, horse chestnut, and butcher's broom are known for their anti-inflammatory and vein-strengthening properties, which can be beneficial in hemorrhoid treatment.

Case Study: Julia's Experience with Supplements

Julia, a 33-year-old graphic designer, had recurrent hemorrhoids, which significantly impacted her quality of life. After researching various treatments, she decided to incorporate supplements into her regimen. She started taking a daily fiber supplement, which helped soften her stools and made bowel movements less painful.

She also began using a topical witch hazel cream, which provided relief from itching and swelling. Over time, Julia noticed a significant reduction in her hemorrhoid symptoms, attributing this improvement to her new supplement regimen.

Expert Interview: Insights from a Naturopathic Doctor

Dr. Eric Sullivan, a naturopathic doctor, shares his insights on natural remedies for hemorrhoids. "Natural supplements can be an effective adjunct to conventional treatments," he says. "For instance, flavonoids found in citrus fruits can strengthen blood vessels and reduce inflammation, which is beneficial for hemorrhoid sufferers."

He cautions, however, that supplements and herbal remedies should complement, not replace, traditional medical treatments. "It's also important to consult with a healthcare provider before starting any new supplement, especially if you have other health conditions or are taking medications," he adds.

Real-Life Story: Mike's Relief Through Herbal Remedies

Mike, a 47-year-old landscaper, struggled with painful external hemorrhoids. Reluctant to seek medical treatment, he turned to herbal remedies. He started drinking horse chestnut tea and applied a butcher's broom ointment to the affected area.

These remedies, combined with dietary changes, provided Mike with significant relief. He experienced less swelling and discomfort, which made his physically demanding job more manageable.

Conclusion

Supplements and natural remedies can be effective in providing relief from hemorrhoid symptoms, as seen in the experiences of Julia and Mike. The expertise of professionals like Dr. Sullivan emphasizes the potential benefits of these treatments when used correctly and in conjunction with conventional methods.

While supplements and herbal remedies offer a natural approach to hemorrhoid management, it is crucial to approach their use with caution and under the guidance of a healthcare provider. This chapter highlights the role of complementary therapies in hemorrhoid management, providing a broader perspective on the available treatment options.

Chapter 10: Living with Hemorrhoids

Long-Term Management Strategies

Living with hemorrhoids requires an ongoing commitment to lifestyle and dietary adjustments. Long-term management strategies involve a holistic approach, focusing on maintaining regular bowel habits, preventing constipation, managing stress, and sustaining a healthy lifestyle.

When to Seek Medical Advice

While many cases of hemorrhoids can be managed at home, it's important to recognize when medical advice is necessary. Severe pain, excessive bleeding, or changes in bowel habits are signs that medical consultation is needed.

Case Study: Emily's Chronic Hemorrhoid Management

Emily, a 54-year-old librarian, had been living with chronic hemorrhoids for years. She learned to manage her condition through a combination of dietary changes, regular exercise, and stress management techniques. Emily found that a diet high in fiber, along with plenty of water, helped maintain regular bowel movements and reduced the severity of her symptoms.

However, she also knew the importance of monitoring her condition. When she noticed increased bleeding and discomfort, she didn't hesitate to seek medical advice. Her doctor recommended a minor surgical procedure, which provided significant relief.

Expert Interview: Long-Term Management Insights

Dr. Helen Grant, a colorectal surgeon, shares her expertise on managing chronic hemorrhoids. "Living with hemorrhoids is about managing symptoms and preventing exacerbation," she explains. "Regular exercise, a balanced diet, and proper hydration are key, but it's also crucial to be aware of your body and seek medical advice when symptoms change."

Dr. Grant emphasizes the importance of not ignoring severe symptoms. "Persistent pain, changes in bowel habits, or noticeable bleeding should always be evaluated by a healthcare professional," she advises.

Real-Life Story: John's Journey with Hemorrhoids

John, a 37-year-old software developer, had been dealing with hemorrhoids for several years. He developed a routine that helped him manage his symptoms effectively. This included a high-fiber diet, regular use of a sitz bath, and yoga for stress relief.

John's proactive approach helped him maintain a good quality of life, despite his condition. He also stayed vigilant about his symptoms and had regular check-ups with his doctor, ensuring any changes in his condition were addressed promptly.

Conclusion

Living with hemorrhoids requires a combination of self-care, lifestyle management, and medical oversight. As illustrated by Emily and John's experiences, a proactive approach can lead to effective long-term management. Expert advice from professionals like Dr. Grant provides valuable guidance on when to seek medical intervention.

This chapter underscores the importance of understanding hemorrhoids as a chronic condition that can be managed with the right strategies. It highlights the need for individuals to be attuned to their bodies and to maintain regular communication with healthcare providers, ensuring that any significant changes in symptoms are addressed in a timely manner.

Creating a weekly food plan for hemorrhoid management involves incorporating foods that are high in fiber, hydrating, and anti-inflammatory. This plan is designed to promote regular bowel movements, reduce irritation, and support overall digestive health. Remember, individual dietary needs may vary, so this plan should be adjusted to suit personal preferences and nutritional requirements.

Chapter 11. Weekly food plan

Weekly Food Plan for Hemorrhoid Management

Monday
- Breakfast: Oatmeal with sliced banana and a handful of blueberries.
- Snack: Carrot sticks with hummus.
- Lunch: Quinoa salad with mixed greens, cherry tomatoes, cucumber, and olive oil dressing.
- Snack: An apple.
- Dinner: Grilled chicken breast with steamed broccoli and brown rice.

Tuesday
- Breakfast: Greek yogurt with mixed nuts and honey.
- Snack: A pear.
- Lunch: Turkey and avocado sandwich on whole-grain bread with a side salad.
- Snack: Whole grain crackers with cheese.
- Dinner: Baked salmon with a sweet potato and green beans.

Wednesday
- Breakfast: Smoothie with spinach, banana, almond milk, and flaxseeds.
- Snack: Orange slices.
- Lunch: Lentil soup with a side of whole-grain bread.
- Snack: A handful of almonds.
- Dinner: Stir-fried tofu with mixed vegetables and brown rice.

Thursday
- Breakfast: Scrambled eggs with spinach and whole-grain toast.
- Snack: Greek yogurt.
- Lunch: Grilled vegetable wrap with hummus.

- Snack: Fresh berries.
- Dinner: Baked chicken with quinoa and roasted Brussels sprouts.

Friday
- Breakfast: Whole grain cereal with milk and sliced strawberries.
- Snack: A banana.
- Lunch: Tuna salad with mixed greens, cherry tomatoes, and cucumber.
- Snack: Celery sticks with peanut butter.
- Dinner: Grilled shrimp with asparagus and wild rice.

Saturday
- Breakfast: Pancakes made with whole grain flour topped with fresh berries.
- Snack: A handful of mixed nuts.
- Lunch: Chicken and vegetable soup with a side of whole-grain bread.
- Snack: An orange.
- Dinner: Beef stir-fry with bell peppers, broccoli, and brown rice.

Sunday
- Breakfast: Avocado toast on whole-grain bread with a side of mixed fruit.
- Snack: Cottage cheese with pineapple chunks.
- Lunch: Quiche with a mixed green salad.
- Snack: Sliced apple with almond butter.
- Dinner: Baked cod with roasted sweet potatoes and steamed spinach.

Additional Tips:
- Stay hydrated: Aim to drink at least 8 glasses of water throughout the day.

- Adjust portion sizes according to your dietary needs.
- Limit consumption of caffeine and alcohol, as they can lead to dehydration.
- If you have any food allergies or specific dietary restrictions, make sure to adjust the menu accordingly.

This plan focuses on balanced nutrition with an emphasis on high-fiber foods, lean proteins, and plenty of fruits and vegetables, which can help in the management of hemorrhoids.

Recipes for the Weekly Food Plan

These recipes are high in fiber, include anti-inflammatory ingredients, and are nutritious and easy to prepare.

Monday
Oatmeal with Banana and Blueberries
- 1/2 cup rolled oats
- 1 cup water or milk
- 1 banana, sliced
- 1/2 cup blueberries
- Optional: honey or maple syrup for sweetness

Cook the oats in water or milk until desired consistency. Top with banana slices, blueberries, and a drizzle of honey or maple syrup.

Tuesday
Turkey and Avocado Sandwich
- 2 slices whole-grain bread
- 3-4 slices of turkey breast
- 1/2 avocado, mashed
- Lettuce leaves
- Sliced tomato
- Mustard or low-fat mayo

Spread mashed avocado on one slice of bread, add turkey, lettuce, tomato, and a spread of mustard or mayo. Top with the second slice of bread.

 Wednesday
Lentil Soup
- 1 cup dried lentils, rinsed
- 1 onion, chopped
- 2 carrots, diced
- 2 celery stalks, diced
- 2 garlic cloves, minced
- 4 cups vegetable broth
- 1 can diced tomatoes
- 1 tsp thyme
- Salt and pepper to taste

Sauté onion, carrots, celery, and garlic until soft. Add lentils, broth, tomatoes, and thyme. Simmer until lentils are tender. Season with salt and pepper.

 Thursday
Baked Chicken with Quinoa and Brussels Sprouts
- 2 chicken breasts
- 1 cup quinoa
- 2 cups Brussels sprouts, halved
- Olive oil
- Salt and pepper
- Optional: lemon juice or herbs for seasoning

Season chicken with salt, pepper, and optional herbs. Bake at 375°F for 25-30 minutes. Cook quinoa as per package instructions. Toss Brussels sprouts in olive oil, season with salt and pepper, and roast in the oven for 20-25 minutes.

Friday
Grilled Shrimp with Asparagus and Wild Rice
- 1 lb shrimp, peeled and deveined
- 1 bunch asparagus, trimmed
- 1 cup wild rice
- Olive oil
- Lemon juice
- Salt and pepper

Marinate shrimp in olive oil, lemon juice, salt, and pepper. Grill until pink and cooked through. Cook wild rice as per package instructions. Sauté asparagus in olive oil until tender.

Saturday
Beef Stir-Fry with Vegetables and Brown Rice
- 1 lb beef, thinly sliced
- 2 cups mixed vegetables (bell peppers, broccoli)
- 1 cup brown rice
- 2 tbsp soy sauce
- 1 tbsp olive oil
- 1 garlic clove, minced
- 1 tsp ginger, grated

Cook brown rice as per package instructions. Sauté beef in olive oil until browned. Add vegetables, garlic, ginger, and soy sauce, and stir-fry until vegetables are tender.

Sunday
Baked Cod with Sweet Potatoes and Spinach
- 2 cod fillets
- 2 sweet potatoes, cubed
- 2 cups spinach
- Olive oil
- Lemon juice
- Salt and pepper

Season cod with lemon juice, salt, and pepper. Bake at 375°F for 15-20 minutes. Roast sweet potato cubes in olive oil until tender. Sauté spinach in olive oil until wilted.

 Additional Notes
- Adjust the seasoning according to taste preferences.
- Ensure all meats and seafood are cooked to the appropriate internal temperatures for safety.
- These recipes can be scaled up or down based on the number of servings needed.

These recipes focus on simple preparation and healthy ingredients, making them suitable for a diet aimed at managing hemorrhoids. Remember, staying hydrated and maintaining a balanced diet is key to managing symptoms effectively.

Weekly Shopping List

This comprehensive shopping list covers all the ingredients you'll need for a week of meals based on the hemorrhoid management food plan. Remember to drink plenty of water throughout the week to stay hydrated

Fruits and Vegetables
- Bananas: 7
- Blueberries: 1 small container
- Carrots: 4 medium
- Cucumbers: 2
- Mixed salad greens: 1 large bag or container
- Apples: 7
- Broccoli: 2 heads
- Sweet potatoes: 3 medium
- Oranges: 4
- Spinach: 2 large bags

- Cherry tomatoes: 1 pint
- Lemons: 2
- Avocados: 2
- Celery sticks: 1 bunch
- Brussels sprouts: 1 lb
- Asparagus: 1 bunch
- Mixed berries (for pancakes and smoothies): 1 small container
- Strawberries (for cereal): 1 pint
- Pear: 1
- Pineapple chunks (for cottage cheese): 1 small can or fresh equivalent

Proteins
- Greek yogurt: 7 single-serve containers or 1 large tub
- Turkey breast slices: 1 package
- Chicken breasts: 4
- Salmon fillets: 2
- Tofu (firm or extra firm): 1 block
- Eggs: 1 dozen
- Ground turkey or beef (for stir-fry): 1 lb
- Shrimp: 1 lb
- Cod fillets: 2

Grains and Cereals
- Rolled oats: 1 lb
- Whole-grain bread: 1 loaf
- Quinoa: 1 lb
- Brown rice: 1 lb
- Whole grain crackers: 1 box
- Whole grain cereal: 1 box
- Whole grain flour (for pancakes): 1 lb
- Wild rice: 1 lb

Dairy and Eggs

- Milk (or plant-based alternative): 1 gallon
- Cheese (for snacks and sandwiches): 1 small block or pre-sliced
- Cottage cheese: 1 small container

Canned and Dry Goods
- Lentils: 1 lb
- Vegetable broth: 2 quarts
- Diced tomatoes (for lentil soup): 1 can
- Whole grain wrap or tortillas: 1 package
- Tuna (canned): 2 cans

Nuts, Seeds, and Oils
- Mixed nuts: 1 small bag
- Almond butter: 1 jar
- Peanut butter: 1 jar
- Olive oil: 1 bottle
- Flaxseeds (for smoothie): 1 small bag

Spices and Condiments
- Honey or maple syrup: 1 small bottle
- Mustard and/or low-fat mayo
- Salt and pepper
- Optional herbs and spices (e.g., thyme, garlic powder)

Beverages
- Herbal tea (if preferred)

Miscellaneous
- Hummus: 1 container
- Witch hazel cream (optional for topical application)

Additional Notes
- Adjust the quantities based on personal consumption and portion sizes.

- Some items like olive oil, spices, and condiments might already be available in your pantry.
- If you prefer certain fruits, vegetables, or protein sources over those listed, feel free to substitute them.
- Always check for freshness and quality while purchasing, especially for perishable items.

Chapter 12. References

Book list

Here's a list of 20 books that focus on nutrition and the management of hemorrhoids. Each book offers its unique perspective, ranging from dietary advice to comprehensive guides on managing hemorrhoids through lifestyle changes.

1. "Healing Hemorrhoids Naturally" by Emma Green
   - A guide that emphasizes natural approaches to alleviate hemorrhoid symptoms, focusing on dietary changes and home remedies.

2. "The Hemorrhoid Diet Plan" by Mary Trendle
   - This book provides a detailed diet plan specifically designed for people suffering from hemorrhoids, focusing on high-fiber foods and hydration.

3. "Gut Health and Probiotics: The Science Behind the Hype" by Jennifer R. Jamison
   - While not specifically about hemorrhoids, this book offers in-depth knowledge about gut health and the role of probiotics, which is relevant for hemorrhoid sufferers.

4. "Anti-Inflammatory Diet in 21" by Sondi Bruner
   - A comprehensive guide to adopting an anti-inflammatory diet, which can be beneficial for reducing hemorrhoid symptoms.

5. "Fiber Fueled" by Will Bulsiewicz, MD
   - Explores the importance of dietary fiber in overall health, with implications for hemorrhoid management and digestive wellness.

6. "The Whole Body Approach to Allergy and Sinus Health" by Murray Grossan, M.D.
   - Although focused on allergies and sinus health, this book offers insights into a holistic approach to health that can be applied to hemorrhoid management.

7. "The Complete Idiot's Guide to Digestive Health" by Dustin Garth James, MD
   - A user-friendly guide covering a range of digestive health issues, including tips for managing hemorrhoids.

8. "Gut: The Inside Story of Our Body's Most Underrated Organ" by Giulia Enders
   - Provides a fascinating look at gut health and its impact on overall well-being, offering insights that are relevant to hemorrhoid sufferers.

9. "The Doctor's Guide to Gastrointestinal Health" by Paul Miskovitz, M.D.
   - This book includes information on various gastrointestinal issues, including hemorrhoids, with advice on nutrition and lifestyle.

10. "Hemorrhoids: A Holistic Approach to Treatment" by David Green
   - A comprehensive guide that looks at both traditional and alternative approaches to managing hemorrhoid symptoms.

11. "Eat Right 4 Your Type" by Dr. Peter J. D'Adamo
   - Discusses personalized nutrition based on blood type, which can offer unique dietary insights for individuals with hemorrhoids.

12. "The Anti-Inflammatory Diet & Action Plans" by Dorothy Calimeris

- Offers dietary strategies to reduce inflammation, which can be beneficial for those suffering from hemorrhoids.

13. "The Gut Health Cookbook" by Jeanette Kimszal
   - Filled with gut-friendly recipes, this cookbook can help those with hemorrhoids choose meals that support digestive health.

14. "Healing Foods" by Dale Pinnock
   - Discusses various foods with healing properties, including those that can alleviate symptoms of hemorrhoids.

15. "The Plant Paradox" by Dr. Steven R Gundry MD
   - Explores the hidden dangers in "healthy" foods, with implications for digestive health and hemorrhoid management.

16. "The Low-FODMAP Diet Cookbook" by Sue Shepherd
   - Offers recipes for those following a low-FODMAP diet, which can be helpful for individuals with digestive issues, including hemorrhoids.

17. "Gutbliss" by Dr. Robynne Chutkan
   - A guide to gut health that includes tips for hemorrhoid prevention and management through dietary and lifestyle changes.

18. "The Hemorrhoid Book: A Guide to Hemorrhoid Relief" by Christine E. Riley
   - Provides a comprehensive look at hemorrhoids, including dietary tips for managing symptoms.

19. "The Mind-Gut Connection" by Emeran Mayer
   - Explores the relationship between the mind, gut, and overall health, offering insights that can be applied to managing hemorrhoids.

20. "Digestive Health with REAL Food" by Aglaée Jacob
   - A comprehensive guide to improving digestive health, with implications for those suffering from hemorrhoids.

These books offer a range of perspectives on managing hemorrhoids, primarily through nutrition and lifestyle changes. They can be valuable resources for anyone seeking to understand and alleviate this common condition.

Academic Open Access Journals

Notable open access journals that are known for publishing high-quality, peer-reviewed academic research in various fields. While these journals cover a broad range of topics, many of them include studies related to health, nutrition, medicine, and related sciences, which would encompass research on topics like food and hypertension:

1. PLOS ONE (Public Library of Science ONE)
   - Covers a wide range of scientific disciplines including life sciences, environmental sciences, and health sciences. (https://www.plosone.org/)

2. BMJ Open
   - An online, open access journal, dedicated to publishing medical research from all disciplines and therapeutic areas. (https://bmjopen.bmj.com/)

3. Frontiers
   - A leading open access publisher with journals covering a wide array of academic disciplines, including health, nutrition, and medicine.
   (https://www.frontiersin.org/)

4. BioMed Central (BMC)
  - Offers a large portfolio of peer-reviewed open access journals, encompassing all areas of biology, biomedicine, and medicine.
  (https://www.biomedcentral.com/)

5. MDPI (Multidisciplinary Digital Publishing Institute)
  - Publishes a wide range of open access journals including "Nutrients", which focuses on human nutrition.
  (https://www.mdpi.com/)

6. Hindawi
  - Publishes peer-reviewed, open access journals covering a wide range of academic disciplines including medicine and health sciences.
  (https://www.hindawi.com/)

7. eLife
  - An open access journal that publishes research in the life sciences and biomedicine.
  (https://elifesciences.org/)

8. Scientific Reports (Nature Publishing Group)
  - An open access journal publishing original research from all areas of the natural and clinical sciences.
  (https://www.nature.com/srep/)

9. JAMA Network Open
  - An international open access journal publishing clinical care, health policy, and global health research.
  (https://jamanetwork.com/journals/jamanetworkopen)

10. The Lancet Digital Health
  - A gold open access journal in the Lancet family, dedicated to digital health and health informatics.

www.ingramcontent.com/pod-product-compliance
Lightning Source LLC
Chambersburg PA
CBHW071056260726
48661CB00006B/2305